Yogic Breathing Techniques

for

Vitality Good Health & Looking Younger

By Subodh Gupta
Corporate Yoga Trainer

First Edition July 2010

ISBN:1453675574
EAN-13: 9781453675571

Subodh Gupta
Head office: London (UK)
Email: info@subodhgupta.com
Website: www.subodhgupta.com
44(0)7966275913

Publisher Note:
The reader should not regard the recommendations and breathing techniques described in this book as substitute advice of a qualified medical practitioner. It is also advisable that reader may learn the breathing exercises initially in the presence of a qualified yoga trainer.

Acknowledgements

I am grateful to my parents and all my teachers who taught me at various stages of my life & shared with me their wisdom.

I am also thankful to the model Shivani Johnsson for taking time out from her busy schedule to help me to complete my book.

Content

Introduction   6

Part 1:

Understanding about breath   9

Type of breath   12

Why the speech of CEO & leaders is thrilling   17

Part 2:

Technique 1: Deep Breathing Exercise   23

Technique 2: Full Yogic Breathing   25

Technique 3: Kapalabhati Exercise   27

Technique 4: Alternate Nostril breathing   33
(Without Breath retention)

Technique 5: Alternate Nostril Breathing   39
(With Breath Retention)

Stress Monitor   47

Practice Record   48

Introduction:

Imagine getting ready for a board meeting or presentation without the natural feelings of tension and anxiety, and having the ability to relax your mind within minutes!

Imagine you can stay energetic and full of energy throughout the day. Imagine that you have the skill to establish yourself in state of tranquillity anytime. Naturally this may seem like a magic trick but the reality is, people who are aware and adept in yogic breathing exercises can easily do this.

You can do it too, because breathing is one physical function which is both involuntary (it happen by itself) and voluntary (it can be control consciously).

Effective breathing is very important and essential for vitality & good health. If you find yourself getting tired easily or stressed, you can improve the situation by breathing exercises and you would be amazed to see how quickly you can improve your stamina and reduce your stress.

This simple and significant insight into the art of breathing was known to scientists of India (discovering the inner dimension of human being) thousands of years ago.

This knowledge and technique of Yogic breathing is explained in this book in a step by step method, along with precautions in the simplest possible way so that everybody can understand and gain benefit.

This book has been divided into 2 sections.

Section 1 contains knowledge and explanation of breath from various perspectives and section 2 includes five practical techniques step by step. It is important to read section 1 first before trying the simple breathing techniques.

At the end of this book I have provided tools for self assessing stress and tracking your progress. It is a good idea to complete these sheets after practicing breathing techniques everyday, to identify the difference over a period of 4 weeks. Please remember that everyday practice is a must, otherwise all theory and no practice would not give you results. If you are practicing everyday in a correct way then positive results will certainly be there.

After the breathing exercises you will definitely feel relaxed and calm. If you feel tired or uncomfortable in any way, you must check that you are practicing in the correct methods.

I wish to all of you reading this book, radiant health and stress free life.

Subodh Gupta

"The flow of breath can give a clear picture about a person's emotional and mental state"

Part 1:

Understanding about Breath

I think that you will agree, that from the day of your birth and until this present moment, you have been constantly breathing without interruption. So let me ask you one question.

How many times do you breathe in a day??? (One breath equals to one inhalation and one exhalation).
..
..
..

..

..

Any ideas? Still thinking ....
Ok, let me give you the answer.

We usually take around 13-15 breaths in a minute. This way if you count, the total numbers of breaths, comes to around 18720 - 21,600 times per day; on average 20000 times in a day.

Yes, you did read correctly, around twenty thousand times in a day! Now you might be thinking why am I asking you such a question. The reason is I would like to emphasise the fact that breathing is one of the most important functions in our body but it is the most neglected one. It influences the activity of each and every cell in our body and most importantly, it is intimately linked with the performance of the brain.

Breath is the life force that sustains life. When the breath stops, life ends. Simple breathing exercises help to control this life force in an extraordinary way and bring tremendous benefits, such as increased energy and perception, and development of the brain.

Normally, most people use only a fraction of their lung capacity for breathing. Shallow breathing deprives the body of oxygen and energy and it leads to disharmony in the body. This results in hunched shoulders and incorrect postures. Many people get tired easily in their daily working schedule and do not realize that this could be corrected by proper breathing exercises. With simple deep and controlled breathing exercises, the absorption of energy can be increased which enhances dynamism and general wellbeing. Awareness and control of the breath also allows us to control our emotions, so proper breathing is a must and required for maintaining good health and liveliness.

Why it is important to develop the awareness of breath and gain conscious control over it?

Our body cannot live without life energy/breath. If our breath is allowed to run on its own, then our unconscious mind controls our breath and the breath is affected (you will notice it when you start observing yourself).

Whenever our state of mind is disturbed then our breath is also disturbed for a long period of time and it is not good for our health in the long run.

However, if we can become aware of our breath, then we can become aware of our mental state. By learning few breathing techniques we can consciously control our breath and can even manage our mental and emotional state instead of being controlled by it.

Link of Breath, Mind and Body

Breath is the link between body and mind; it can be regulated by the mind or it can be left to the body. Although breath is not controlled by either of them exclusively, it can be affected by both of them and in turn is the key to the interaction of body and mind.

Breath and Emotions:

There is a direct relationship between the breath of a person and his / her emotional state.

Flow of breath can give a clear picture about a person's emotional and mental state. When the breath is relaxed and slow it gives an indication of calmness, however, if the breath is uneven and disrupted it gives an indication of emotional and mental disturbance.

Breath can be agitated if the person is angry, it can be stopped momentarily in cases of fear, it can be choked in sadness and sighing with relief.

Physical exercise can affect the emotional state of person and so does his/ her breath.

The emotional and mental state of a person are difficult factors to control, however they are linked with breath, and breath can be controlled, i.e. emotional and mental state of human being can be controlled by controlling breath.

Type of Breath

For simplicity of reading, I have avoided going much into technical terminology regarding breathing and have chosen breath patterns from practical point of view which everybody can easily understand. There are 4 different ways in which people breathe in their daily life:

(a) Clavicular breathing

(b) Thoracic Breathing / Chest Breathing

(c) Paradoxical Breathing

(d) Deep Abdominal Breathing / Diaphragmatic breathing

Clavicular breathing is the most shallow and least effective breathing. Its name derives from the two clavicles (collarbones) that are pulled upwards when you complete your inhalation.

With this breathing method *shoulders and collarbone area are raised*, and *abdomen is contracted* during inhalation.

In this type of breathing one has to apply the maximum effort to breathe in and a minimum amount of air is inhaled.

We get very little energy from the atmosphere in this type of breath. In day to day life, clavicular breathing is rarely used except under extreme conditions.

Thoracic breathing or Chest Breathing is done with the rib muscles expanding the rib cage.

This breathing is usually shallow and rapid. This technique fills the middle and upper portion of lungs with air, however it is not good enough for the lower portion. If you are in a standing position, most of the blood will be in the lower area of the lungs because of gravity so the gas exchange which takes place between air in the lungs and blood would not be complete.

This is the type of breathing which is often associated with physical exercises and stress/ tension. I have seen this mostly in gym enthusiasts who tend to use this breathing technique. However, people continue this kind of breathing even after they come out of gym which results in a unhealthy breathing habit.

This breathing is better than Clavicular, although still not a complete method because the amount of air inhaled is less than that when compare to deep abdominal breathing.

It also results in more work for the heart, when compared to diaphragmatic breathing, because chest breathing requires comparatively more work for blood and gases to mix, so more oxygen is needed. This results in more breaths and to get more breaths more blood is need to circulate which finally results in more work for the heart.

Also in my Yogic experience, I have observed that thoughts of anxiety are more associated with chest breathing as compared to deep abdominal / diaphragmatic breathing.

So the simple analysis is, *if you want your heart to do less work, chest breathing or thoracic breathing is not the best method.*

Paradoxical Breathing

This type of breathing pattern involves a combination of *expanding the chest* and *contracting the abdominal muscles* during the *inhalation* process. In this breathing, although the chest wall expands and lung volume is increased, however, the diaphragm simultaneously rises and reduces the gain of increase lung volume.

This breathing pattern is called Paradoxical breathing because the *abdominal wall moves in rather than out during inhalation* and *out rather than in during exhalation process.*

I am surprised to have seen many times in my yoga classes, that beginners use this kind of breathing because it has become their habit.

I cannot stress enough that this is not the efficient way to breathe.

Deep abdominal breathing or **diaphragmatic breathing** is the best among all of the breathing patterns.

In this breathing exercise *during inhalation*, the *diaphragm moves downward*. This pushes the *abdominal down and outward*. During *exhalation*, the *diaphragm moves upward* and the *abdomen moves inward*.

In this type of breathing we extract more energy from our breath as compared to the other two types of breath and it is the most natural and efficient way to breathe. Diaphragmatic breathing can be practiced either in a standing position or a sitting position, or even in a lying position on your back.

In my experience, if you can practice consciously slow and deep diaphragmatic breathing every day, you will feel the noticeable improvement in your state of mind and certainly you will find freedom from anxiety, stress and hypertension.

Why abdominal breathing (diaphragmatic breathing) is the most natural and efficient way to breathe?

There are many reasons for using the Diaphragmatic Breathing:

The lungs are pear shaped, with the narrow end pointing

upwards. This means that with *chest breathing,* only the narrow top part of the lungs are used, rather than the *larger deeper recesses accessed during diaphragmatic breathing.*

In Diaphragmatic breathing, expansion is focused on the lower area of the lungs (there is more blood in the lower area of each lung because of gravity) where oxygen exchange can take place more efficiently with blood.

With each diaphragmatic breath the abdominal organs are massaged, they are stimulated and invigorated. This alternating squeezing and relaxing action helps to pump the blood through the organs of the abdomen and helps in moving waste through the intestines.

Less energy is required to breathe with the diaphragm muscle *than* with the chest muscles. Shallow chest breathing never empties the waste products from the deep recesses of your lungs where they accumulate and stagnate. *Whenever possible breathe diaphragmatically.*

Yogic Breath

Deep breathing exercise is recommended in day to day life as a healthy breathing method however, none of the above breathing patterns are complete.
A complete breathing process is full yogic breath which combines three breathing exercises (abdominal, chest & clavicular) and everyday practice of this method in addition to slow, deep, abdominal breath certainly help in reducing stress and depression, and aid relaxation.

A full yogic breath begins with deep abdominal breathing

and a continuation of the inhalation process through the rib cage and shoulder area. This breathing helps a person to store abundant energy within the body and allow them to work for the whole day and still experience by the end of the day that they are full of energy.

The yogic breathing can be performed everyday for a short time as breathing exercises.

Why the speech of CEO & leaders is so thrilling?

Have you ever wondered why when giving a speech, one speaker may thrill the audience, while the other may have very little or no effect even though they may speak in same style.

The difference is the speech of the first speaker is charged with high energy.

All of the famous leaders you may find in history and in the present time, have wonderful high energy levels and when they speak, people find them inspiring.

Full yogic breathing helps by increasing vitality and your energy levels.

Anyone, with regular practice, can start to see the results within 4 to 6 weeks. The important thing is correct practice and consistency. The ill effects of tension and depression can be overcome or to a great extent reduced by this breathing technique.

Lifestyle, Body Energy Level and Breath

The flow of energy in your body is affected by your lifestyle such as physical activities, work, sleep, food and sex. Your emotions, imagination or thoughts can affect the energy of your body even more. Stress also depletes the energy flow and you may experience feeling totally drained of energy.

The breath is the most vital process of your body. If a person is engaged in deep thinking, relaxation or meditation, the breathing will be slow and steady. If the person is affected by negative emotions, the breathing will become fast, unsteady and irregular. The slow and deep breathing method is very important for increasing the human life span.

If you observe an animal's life span, you can notice that the animals with slow breath rate (elephants, tortoises, pythons) have a longer life span than the one with a fast breathing rate (dogs, rabbits) which live only for few years.

A slow breathing rate keeps the heart stronger and better nourished and leads to a longer life. By breathing slowly and deeply we increase the absorption of energy, enhance our vitality and general wellbeing.

Part 2:

Practical Breathing Techniques

When the body and mind are constantly overworked their natural efficiency decreases. A few moments of stress i.e. anger, anxiety or irritation can consume a great amount of energy leaving the person drained in their daily life.

Psychosomatic illnesses such as diabetes, hypertension, migraine, etc arise from stress. If the mind is tense, the stomach will also be tense, and consequently leave the circulatory system tense.

However, if we are able to reduce our stress levels, we can avoid most of the present-day life style diseases and can enjoy a healthy body and mind.

Have you ever noticed that from time to time after long hours of sleep, you wake up feeling exhausted and you wonder why? The answer is simple. Unless you are free from stress, your body and mind will always be tense and you can never feel relaxed.

However the good news is, we can come out of stress at our own will and our body and mind can be reenergized by the simple breathing exercises.

Before practicing the breathing exercises it is important to consider the following guidelines;

Notes for the practitioners of breathing exercise:

Breathing through nose or mouth: Always breathe through the nose with awareness (unless the yoga teacher specify to breathe through your mouth). *Remember this simple concept that by nature, the mouth is for eating and the nose is for breathing.* Please do not try to reverse nature's functions. As you breathe in, know that you are breathing in. As you breathe out, know that you are breathing out. This will greatly enhance your general health and well-being.

To enlighten you further, the nose doesn't simply allow you to breathe but it also filters the air, moisturises the air, warms the air, it can smell, it secretes mucus and performs many more functions. Now think for a moment, can the mouth perform all of these functions?...

Yes you are thinking correctly, the mouth cannot perform all of these functions, so please do not breathe through the mouth unless specified in some special exercises.

Timing of breathing practices: Simple, slow, and deep breathing exercises (Technique no 1) can be done any time, However Kapalabhati and Alternate Nostril breathing exercises can be done early in the morning for best results or just after sunset. Please remember to breathe in and out slowly when performing techniques no 1, 2, 4 and 5.

Place of practice: It is good to practice in a room which is well ventilated. Please do not practice under a fan or in direct sunlight.

Sitting Posture: Any comfortable sitting position is OK. The main point is the body needs to be relaxed and the back straight. Do not slump and do not lean forward. It is good to sit on a folded blanket or cloth which is made from natural fibre.

Empty stomach: When practice Kapalabhati and Alternate Nostril Breathing exercises please make sure that your stomach is empty, i.e. your last meal should be around 3 and half hour before.

Straining while holding the breath: I have seen many times that participants often try to stain themselves, particularly when holding the breath so that they can advance further (Technique 5).

I repeat again, please never strain your lungs while holding your breath (in technique 5), when doing the practice of alternate nostril breathing as lungs are delicate organs. Forcefully holding the breath beyond your comfort level would only injure your lungs.

Some Symptoms:

It sometimes happens that when you start with regular practice of alternate nostril exercise with breath retention, (technique no 5) that you may experience constipation. If this does happens then please ensure that you drink plenty of water (8 to 10 glasses) per day.

Breath retention and Kapalabhati exercise should not be practiced when you feel unwell.

Breath is life itself and each incoming breath brings the gift of life, and each out flowing breath can be a natural release of tension and negativity.

Breathing Technique no 1

Diaphragmatic Breathing

Deep abdominal breathing or diaphragmatic breathing happens because of action of the diaphragm.

In this breathing exercise, *during inhalation,* the *diaphragm moves downward,* and pushes the *abdominal down and outward.* During *exhalation,* the *diaphragm moves upward* and the *abdomen moves inward.*

Abdominal breathing is the most natural and efficient breathing method. One can observe a little baby breath since the moment of his/her birth and it is diaphragmatic breathing only.

When performing and learning abdominal breathing
First lie down flat on your back, and relax your whole body. Check yourself to see if there is tension in any of your body parts, and if you find any tightness just release it. Now direct your awareness towards your breath.

Next, observe your natural breath, making sure that you are not controlling it but only observing it.

Now, place your left hand on the abdomen on your navel area.

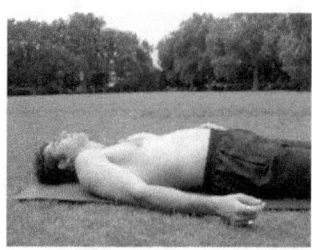

(Position of abdomen during inhalation)

If you are breathing naturally through your abdomen, your left hand (which is above the abdomen) would *move up with inhalation* and *down with exhalation*.

Try to take your breath deeper and deeper into the lungs, so that you feel the abdomen lifting as you breathe in and falling as you breathe out.

Gradually you will notice that the abdomen is moving more firmly, and the chest is moving less. As abdominal breathing becomes easier to you, try to let your breathing become *slower, deeper* and *smoother*.

This slow, deep and smooth breath will bring relaxation to the body and mind. This is the breathing pattern you can use all the times, while at rest or at work. Practice it until it becomes natural and unconscious.

Cautions:
Make sure that there are no jerks in flow of your breath. The flow of your breath should be smooth and without any noise.

Technique no 2

Full yogic breath

Full yogic breath combines the three breathing techniques. In yogic breath, inhalation happens in three stages. However this is done in a smooth way i.e. it looks as if it is a single attempt to breathe in without any jerk.

This type of breathing is very helpful in calming the nervous system and releasing stress.

Yogic breath technique step by step:

You can sit in a comfortable posture or lie down in the relaxation posture called savasana whichever position you prefer.

Observe your breath just outside your nostril area for about the next ten breaths.

Now inhale slowly and deeply (*abdominal breathing*) and when you feel that abdomen has comfortably expanded enough, *then* try expending the chest area by expanding the ribs. *After* the ribs are expended comfortably, try inhaling a little more air to expand the upper portion of the lungs and base of the neck. In this process, shoulders and collar bones will also move up a little.

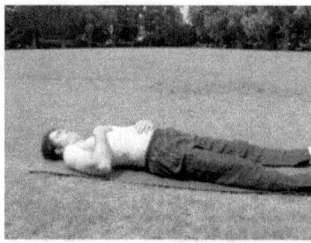

Now start to exhale slowly, relaxing the lower neck and upper chest area, then the chest and finally the abdomen which you will feel coming in. Try to exhale completely by pulling the abdominal muscles in within your comfort level.

One inhalation and one exhalation, is equal to one breath or one round of yogic breath. You can practice 10 rounds every day.

Cautions:
Make sure that there are no jerks in the flow of your breath. The flow of your breath should be smooth and without any noise.

Technique no 3

Kapalabhati exercise

(Cleansing Breathing Exercise)

Kapala in Sanskrit means *skull* and Bhati means *shining*. Practicing kapalabhati on a regular basis leads to a shining skull and face, beaming with good health.

Kapalabhati is a highly energizing abdominal breathing exercise. It cleans the respiratory passage and stimulates the digestive organs.

Beginners can begin this exercise method in its mild form i.e. do not push your abdomen too much while exhaling.

What we do in Kapalabhati

In Kapalabhati we do *quick* exhalation and *natural* inhalation. Normally exhalation takes one fourth of the time of inhalation.

Quick exhalation and natural inhalation follow each other. This cycle of quick exhalation and natural inhalation is repeated several times.

How to do Kapalabhati

Step 1) Sit in a comfortable crossed leg position with the back straight. Hands comfortably resting on knees. Face to be relaxed.

Step 2) Inhale deeply through both nostrils, expanding the abdomen.

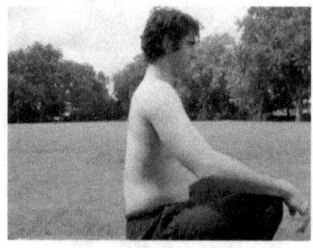

Step 3) Now, exhale with the *forceful contraction* of the abdominal muscles. (*Pull the abdomen in by quickly contracting the abdominal muscles and exhale through the nose*).

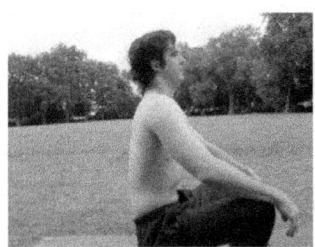

Model Duncan Hogg

The air is pushed out of the lungs by contraction of the diaphragm.

Step 4) After exhalation you should inhale again, but *this inhalation should not involve any effort.*

To inhale, just relax and the lungs will automatically expand and fill with air. You can begin with 10 respirations. After completing 10 quick exhalations and natural inhalations, relax and breathe naturally. This is one round. You can start the practice of Kapalabhati with 3 rounds.

Benefits of Kapalabhati
1) Kapalabhati cleanses the lungs and the entire respiratory system.
2) The blood is purified and the body gets an increased supply of oxygen to all cells.

3) Digestion is improved.
4) Abdominal muscles are strengthened.
5) Prepares the mind for meditation.
6) Energises the mind for mental work.

Precautions:

Kapalabhati should not be practiced by those suffering from the following:

a) Heart disease
b) High blood pressure
c) Hernia
d) Vertigo
e) When Asthmatic attack in progress.

f) If pain or dizziness is experienced *it is preferable to stop the practice till the sensation has passed. Practice can then be restarted with less force.*

g) Quick exhalation should be comfortable and *should not be too forceful.*

h) In you are pregnant you should not practice Kapalabhati.

Common Mistakes:

1) The abdomen is contracted while inhaling. *This mistake is done most often by people* who are habitual *of breathing mostly through chest or paradoxical breathing.*

2) Shoulders are contracted to push the air out when exhaling.

3) Back and shoulders move during exercise.

Point to Note:

a) Exercise should not be done if you feel discomfort at anytime, anywhere in the body during the exercise.

b) Rapid breathing used in this technique should be from the *abdomen* and not from the chest.

c) Kapalabhati should be practiced on an *empty stomach* only.

d) Ideally when doing this exercise along with yoga and meditation, Kapalabhati should be practiced after the yoga postures and relaxation, wait *at least 10 minutes* and before meditation.

e) *People with poor lung capacity should be very careful* whilst doing this exercise and please do not exhale forcefully.

f) The chest should not move very much.

g) *I recommend that in the beginning one should learn this exercise with yoga teacher only.*

"Emotional and mental state of person are difficult to control, however they are linked with breath and breath can be controlled i.e. emotional and mental state of human being can be controlled by controlling breath"

Technique no 4:

Alternate Nostril Breathing
(Without breath retention)

A normal person breathe *predominantly* through *one nostril at a time* i.e. either through right nostril or left nostril and the flow of breath *changes* every 2 to 3 hours from one nostril to another.

Left hemisphere of the brain controls the right side of the body and predominantly involved in logical thinking, analysis and mathematical functions. So when right nostril is clear and freely flowing, in that case right side of body is predominant (and left hemisphere of the brain).

The right hemisphere of brain controls left part of the body and is involved in more creative and artistic functions. And when left nostril is clear, in this case left part of the body is dominant (and right hemisphere of the brain).

If one nostril remains open for several hours without changing the flow to other nostril, this is a sign of some imbalance.

If only one nostril remains active or predominant throughout the day i.e. 24 hours, this is a sign that illness may pursue or already in progress.

Simple Alternate Nostril Breathing exercise helps in establishing the natural rhythm of breath and regular practice help human being in attaining healthy physical and mental state.

Any disease in a body is a sign of imbalance in body's energy level. This simple Alternate Nostril Breathing exercise brings balance in the body energy level and helps the body to remain disease free along with calmness.

Alternate Nostril Breathing (*Without breath retention*) purifies the energy channels in the body which carries the increased energy to some areas of the brain.

It is very important that the channels be purified first to cope with the increased energy created by *advance breathing* exercise of *breath retention*.

It is preferable to close your eyes during practice of Alternate Nostril Breathing.

How to do Alternate Nostril Breathing: (*Without*** *breath retention*)**

1. Inhale completely through the left nostril, keeping the right nostril closed with the right thumb. This can be done by counting up to "4" mentally.

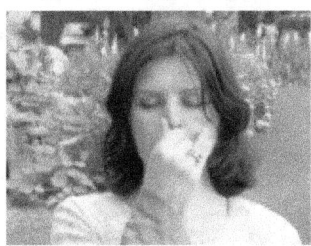

2. Release the right nostril and exhale completely to a count of "4", counting mentally (Close left nostril).

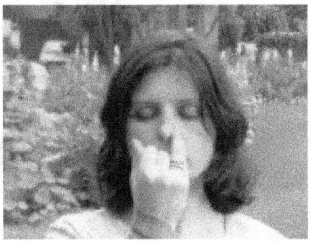

3. Inhale fully through the right nostril to a count of "4". (Left nostril closed).

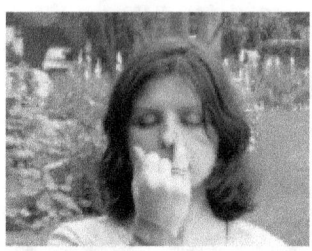

4. Release the left nostril and exhale completely to a count of "4" (Right nostril closed).

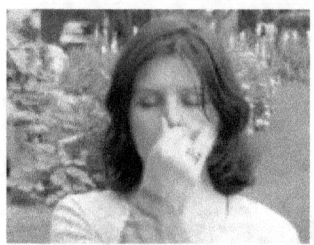

This is one round. At least 20 rounds should be practiced daily and gradually increased to 40 rounds.

Next step after you master this ratio:

After 8 to 12 weeks of regular practice depending upon your comfort level, the "count" of the exercise may be increased.

For example, inhaling to the count of 5 and then exhaling to the count of 5.

After completing this breathing exercise it is good to relax for about 5 to 10 minutes.

By nature

"Mouth is for eating

And

Nose is for breathing"

Technique no 5

Alternate Nostril Breathing
(With breath retention)

This is a advance breathing exercise and should *only* be practiced under the guidance of a experienced yoga trainer.

Sit in any comfortable position. You can sit in any position in which you are comfortable and can sit for about 10 to 15 minutes without any discomfort.

You also have the option to sit on a chair which has straight back or may sit with the support of wall in case if you cannot sit with back straight.

The main point is *comfortable position* and *straight back* with relax body. Observe your breath for about 2 min or say around 25 -30 breaths.

Preparing for Alternate Nostril Breathing exercise (with breath retention)

Raise the right hand. Make the Vishnu Mudra by folding down the index and middle fingers as shown below.

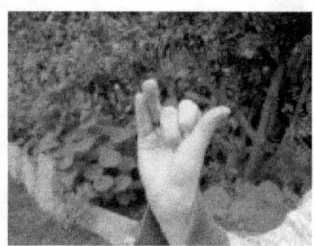

How to do Alternate Nostril Breathing:

1. Inhale completely through the left nostril, keeping the right nostril closed with the right thumb (as shown in picture below). This can be done by counting up to "4" mentally.

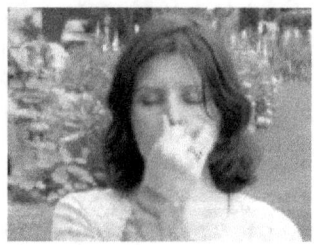

2. Close the left nostril with the *two end* fingers so that both the nostrils are closed (as shown in the picture below). Retain the breath to a count of "4" counting mentally.

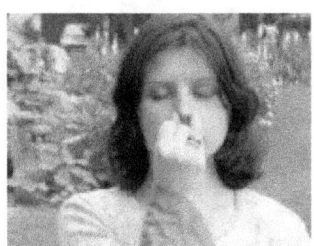

3. Release the right nostril and exhale completely to a count of "4", counting mentally as shown in picture below.

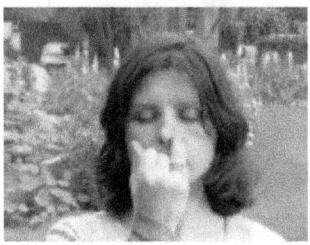

4. Inhale fully through the right nostril to a count of "4" (as shown in the picture below).

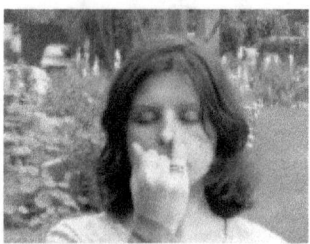

5. Both nostrils closed and retain the breath to a count of "4".

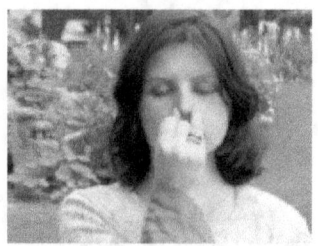

6. Release the left nostril and exhale completely to a count of "4" as shown in the picture below.

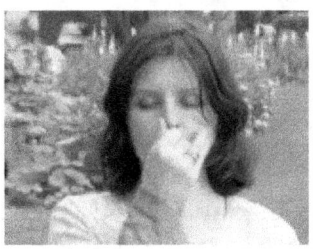

This is one round.
At least 10 rounds should be practiced daily.

Next step

After 8 to 12 weeks of regular practice, depending upon your comfort level the "count" of the exercise may be increased.

For example it can be, inhaling to the count of 5, then retaining the breath to the count of 5 and then releasing the breath to the count of 5.

Next step:

After you master this ratio of 1:1:1 (*i.e. inhaling the breath to the count of 5, retaining breath to the count of 5 and exhaling the breath to the count of 5*), one can increase the ratio to 1:1:2 (*Inhaling to the count of 5, retaining the breath to the count of 5 and exhaling the breath to the count of 10*).

Next Step:
After mastering the ratio of 1:1:2 increase the ratio to 1:2:2. (Inhale the breath to the count of 5, retain the breath to the count of 10 and exhale to the count of 10).

Next Step:
After mastering the ratio of 1:2:2 increase this ratio to 1:3:2 and finally 1:4:2.

Once you reach to the ratio of 1:4:2 then stick to this ratio. For example: you inhale for 4 seconds; you retain the breath for 16 seconds and exhale for 8 seconds , never change the ratio. You may also increase the number of rounds of Alternate Nostril Breathing.

Benefits of Alternate Nostril Breathing (breath retention)
Physical benefits

1. Alternate Nostril Breathing cleanses and strengthens the lungs and entire respiratory system.

2. During retention, there is the highest rate of gaseous exchange in the lungs. Because of the increase in the pressure, more oxygen goes from the lungs into the blood and more CO_2 and other waste products pass from the blood into the lungs for elimination during exhalation.

3. As exhalation is twice the time of inhalation, stale air and waste products are drained from the lugs.

4. This breathing exercise is good for people who are suffering from low blood pressure.

Mental Psychic benefits:

1. Alternate Nostril Breathing helps to calm the mind, making it lucid and steady.

2. It makes the body light and the eyes shiny.

Common Mistakes:

1. Back is not straight.
2. The breath is not smooth.

Precautions:

(1) I would like to repeat here, that *it is* **strongly advised** *that this exercise should only be learnt from an experienced yoga teacher* and not on your own or by watching TV channels or DVD.

(2) **Beginners** should not try this exercise of breath retention instead they can try simple Alternate Nostril Breathing _without_ breath retention.

(3)Please **do not try to hold breath** beyond *your comfort level* as it will not benefit you rather can hurt you as lungs are delicate organs.

(4) People who are suffering from eye or ear problem (like glaucoma or pus in the ear) can be more cautious and preferably do not hold breath.

(5) Please ensure that during practice of *breath retention*, you should not feel any strain in eyes, ears, thighs and arms.

(6)Do not tense your arm while practicing this exercise. Quite often beginners tense their arm.

(7) The place for breathing exercises should be well ventilated.

(8) If you are suffering from high blood pressure or heart trouble, you may please *avoid* this exercise instead practice simple alternate breathing without breath retention.

Stress Monitor

Before beginning breathing exercise plan, please take couple of minutes to fill in the following stress monitor.

	Stress Monitor	
S.N.	Indicators	Before Beginning
1	Blood Pressure (High)	
	(Low)	
2	Hours of sleep (average per week)	
3	Quality of sleep (1 to 5) (1 lowest and 5 the best, average for the week)	
4	Stress level (1 to 5) (1 lowest and 5 highest, average for the week)	
5	Overall energy level (1 to 5) (1 lowest and 5 highest)	

Practice Record

Starting Date......................................

S.N	Week 1	Sun	Mon	Tue	Wed	Thu	Fri	Sat
S.N	Breathing Technique							
1	Simple slow &Deep Abdominal Breathing							
2	Full Yogic Breath							
3	Kapalabhati							
4	Alternate Nostril Breathing (without breath retention)							

After week 1 please record below, how do you feel / improvement

Practice Record

	Week 2	Sun	Mon	Tue	Wed	Thu	Fri	Sat
S.N	Breathing Technique							
1	Simple slow &Deep Abdominal Breathing							
2	Full Yogic Breath							
3	Kapalabhati							
4	Alternate Nostril Breathing (without breath retention)							

After week 2 please record below, how do you feel / improvement

Practice Record

	Week 3	Sun	Mon	Tue	Wed	Thu	Fri	Sat
S.N	Breathing Technique							
1	Simple slow &Deep Abdominal Breathing							
2	Full Yogic Breath							
3	Kapalabhati							
4	Alternate Nostril Breathing (without breath retention)							

After week 3 please record below, how do you feel / improvement

Practice Record

	Week 4	Sun	Mon	Tue	Wed	Thu	Fri	Sat
S.N	Breathing Technique							
1	Simple slow &Deep Abdominal Breathing							
2	Full Yogic Breath							
3	Kapalabhati							
4	Alternate Nostril Breathing (without breath retention)							

After week 4 please record below, how do you feel / improvement

Stress Monitor

After 4 weeks of regular practice of breathing exercise, please take couple of minutes to fill in the following stress monitor.

	Stress Monitor	
S.N.	Indicators	After 4 week
1	Blood Pressure (High)	
	(Low)	
2	Hours of sleep (average per week)	
3	Quality of sleep (1 to 5) (1 lowest and 5 the best, average for the week)	
4	Stress level (1 to 5) (1 lowest and 5 highest, average for the week)	
5	Overall energy level (1 to 5) (1 lowest and 5 highest)	

Dear practitioner,

Please note that you can begin with only the *first two breathing methods* initially and later on you can incorporate exercise number third and fourth in your schedule, if your time permits.

Breathing exercise number five is more for information purpose and should only be tried after couple of months of practicing exercise number four and that too under the guidance of an experienced yoga teacher.

While practicing breathing exercises if you come across any question, you are welcome to send me your query at: Email: info@subodhgupta.com

More information about us is available at www.subodhgupta.com

I wish you good health and happiness in your life.

With Best Wishes
Subodh Gupta

Gentle Yoga for 50 Plus

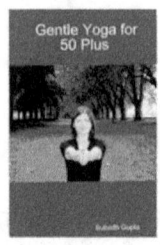

"A perfect <u>gift</u> of health <u>for your parents</u>"

The only book on Gentle Yoga for people in the age group of 50 plus. The exercises explained in this book are also beneficial if suffering from arthritis or rheumatism.

Paperback/ £5.95/ 68 pages

7 Food Habits for Weight Loss *Forever*

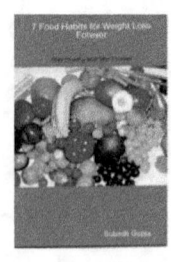

Stay Healthy and Slim *Forever*

"For anybody who wants to lose weight and gain health forever"

"Managing perfect body weight is not a complicated rocket science. Our body is made up of food which we eat during our day to day life. If we are overweight or obese at the moment then one thing is certain that the food which we eat is not good."

Healthy Food Habits = Good Health + Perfect Body Weight *Forever*

ISBN 978-0-9556882-0-1
Page 68 / Soft Cover / £4.95

All our books are available at leading online stores.

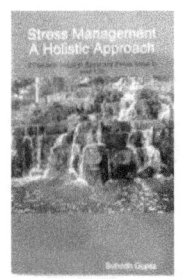

Stress Management a Holistic Approach

5 Steps plan to manage any Stress issue in your life

Many illnesses such as diabetes, migraine, asthma, ulcer and even cancer arise because of excessive Stress over the period of time.

You may have any kind of problem or issue in your life, once you follow the 5 steps described in this book you are on your way to Stress free life. If there is a problem then there has to be a solution and this book is all about solution.

ISBN 978-0-9556882-1-8
Page 80 / Soft Cover / £4.95

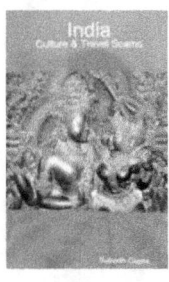

India Culture and Travel scams

"The only book on travel scams targeted at western tourists in India"

This is a practical book about understanding Indian culture and travel scams in India and is based on real life experiences.

This book will help you to avoid embarrassing mistakes and prepare you to feel confident in unfamiliar situations.

Content in this book includes Indian social customs, their perception about Western women, their religion, what motivates them, travel scams targeted at Western tourists and of course what not to discuss with Indians, etc.

Page 112/Paper Back / £7.95
ISBN 978-0-9556882-6-3